Yoga Yin

Cultivating

INNER STRENGTH AND FLEXIBILITY

Dr. Jilesh

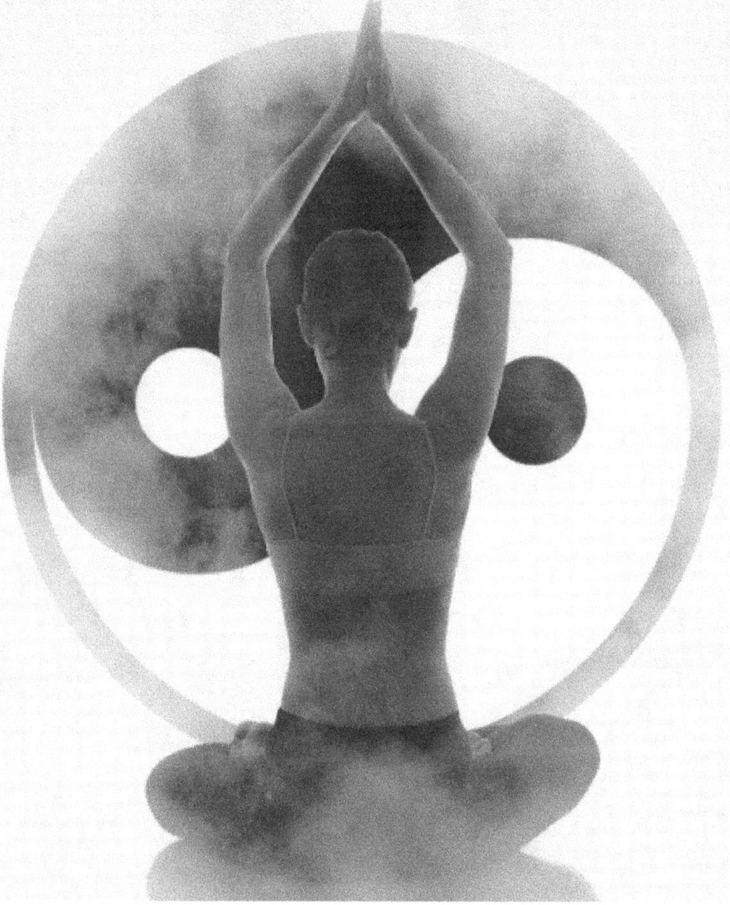

Copyright © 2023 by Jilesh Thilakan

For permissions requests, write to the publisher at the address below:

Publisher: Jilesh Thilakan, India

Website: www.healingoraclewisdom.com[1]

Email: drjilesht@gmail.com

Cover design by Jilesh Thilakan

Disclaimer: The information provided in this book is for general informational purposes only. The content is based on the topic of Yin yoga and aims to explore techniques for cultivating inner strength and flexibility. Yin yoga is a gentle and introspective practice, and individual results may vary. The author and publisher disclaim any liability for any loss or damage incurred by the reader or any third party directly or indirectly as a result of the use or application of the information presented in this book.

The content provided in this book should not be misconstrued as medical or professional advice. Readers seeking specific information about their physical or mental health should consult with qualified healthcare professionals.

---

1. http://www.healingoraclewisdom.com/

The author encourages readers to approach the practice of Yin yoga with mindfulness, self-compassion, and a focus on their unique journey of self-discovery and self-care.

About Author

Dr. Jilesh is a highly accomplished professional with expertise spanning diverse fields, making a profound impact on lives worldwide.

As an Instructor on Udemy, his courses are known for their simplicity and engagement, equipping students with valuable skills. Beyond teaching, he is a compassionate Psychotherapist, supporting individuals in overcoming challenges and fostering emotional well-being.

His Master of Business Administration (MBA) complements his academic and therapeutic pursuits, offering a strategic edge to his endeavours. Moreover, Dr. Jilesh's distinction as a Reiki Grand Master showcases his proficiency in energy healing, providing alternative paths to wellness.

Embracing a holistic approach to personal growth, Dr. Jilesh empowers others to flourish intellectually, emotionally, spiritually, and professionally. A lifelong learner, he continually seeks knowledge to stay at the forefront of education, therapy, business, and energy healing.

An inspiring speaker and advocate, Dr. Jilesh spreads awareness about mental health, the importance of education, and the transformative power of energy healing. His dedication to empowering others reflects his commitment to creating a positive impact on individuals and communities alike.

Introduction

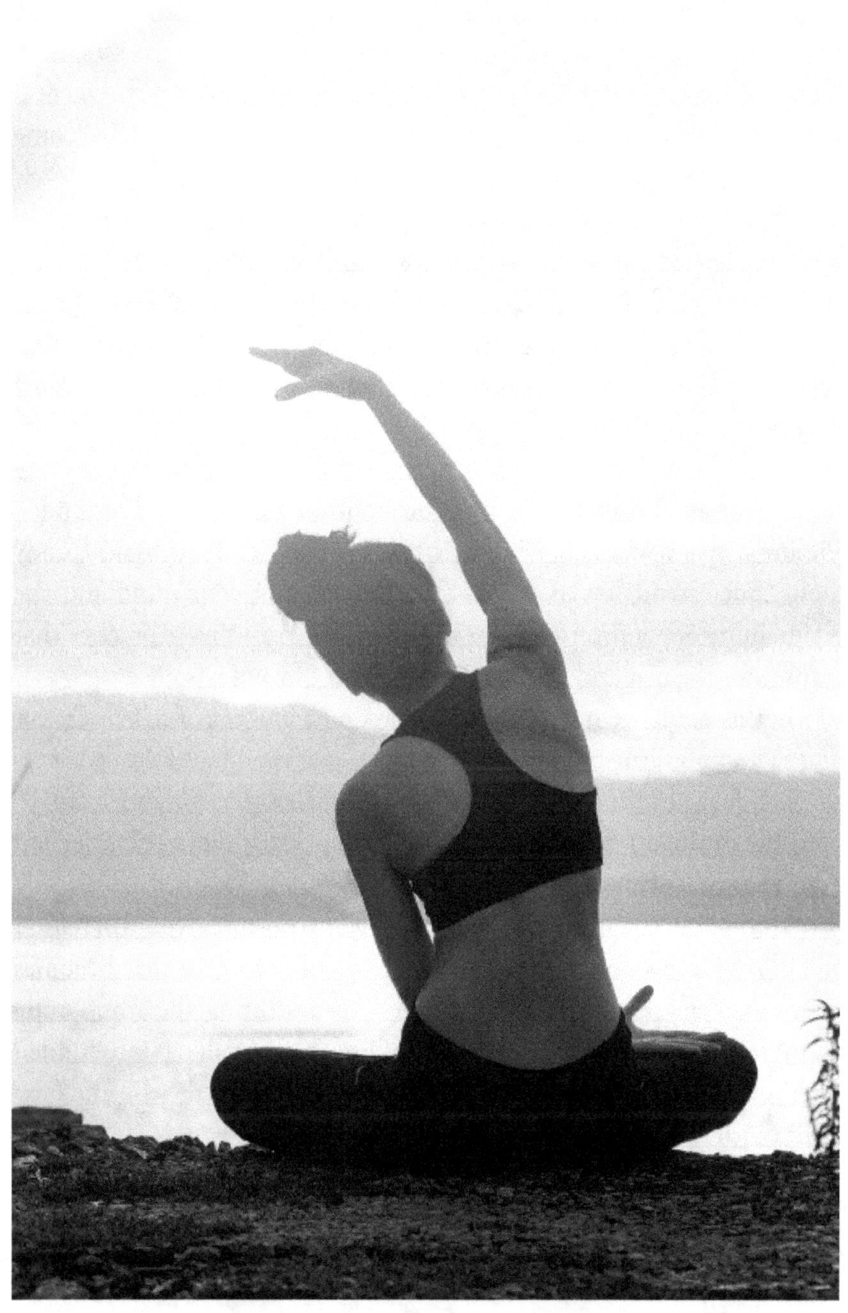

In the hustle and bustle of our modern lives, we often find ourselves caught in the whirlwind of responsibilities, stress, and constant movement. Amidst this chaos, have you ever longed for a sanctuary - a tranquil space where you can reconnect with your inner self, find serenity, and emerge stronger, more flexible, and empowered? Welcome to the transformative world of Yoga Yin.

Yoga Yin: Cultivating Inner Strength and Flexibility is an immersive journey that beckons you to step away from the noise and into the profound realm of Yin Yoga. Beyond the flashy poses and fast-paced flows, lies a hidden gem of gentle, yet deeply impactful practice that can revolutionize your approach to physical, mental, and emotional well-being.

Imagine a yoga practice where the focus is not on pushing boundaries and breaking limits, but on embracing stillness and surrender. Picture a space where flexibility is not confined to the physical body alone, but extends to encompass the resilience of your mind and the adaptability of your spirit. This is the essence of Yoga Yin - a practice that transcends the mat and permeates every facet of your existence.

In this book, we invite you to embark on a journey of self-discovery and self-empowerment like no other. Here, you will unravel the mysteries of Yin Yoga, explore the depths of mindful awareness, and learn to cultivate profound inner strength and flexibility that radiates far beyond your yoga practice.

Through the gentle art of surrendering into postures, you will release the grip of stress and anxiety, fostering a sense of peace that becomes your sanctuary amidst life's challenges. By nurturing the mind-body connection and harnessing the power of breath, you will tap into hidden reservoirs of resilience, empowering yourself to navigate the ebb and flow of life with newfound ease.

Beyond just physical flexibility, you will discover how to embrace change and transformation with an open heart, understanding that growth often springs from the most unexpected places. From the cushioned cocoon of Yin Yoga, you will emerge a butterfly, ready to spread your wings and take flight, embarking on a journey of limitless possibilities.

Whether you are a seasoned yogi or a curious beginner, this book extends its hand to guide you on a path of holistic well-being, bridging the gap between body, mind, and soul. The wisdom and insights shared here will empower you to integrate the tranquillity of Yin Yoga into your daily life, allowing you to

approach challenges with grace, face uncertainties with courage, and embrace the beauty of the present moment with profound gratitude.

So, are you ready to step into the transformative world of Yoga Yin and embark on a journey of inner strength and flexibility? Turn the page, and let the adventure begin. The path to serenity and self-empowerment awaits.

Chapter 1
The Foundations of Yoga Yin

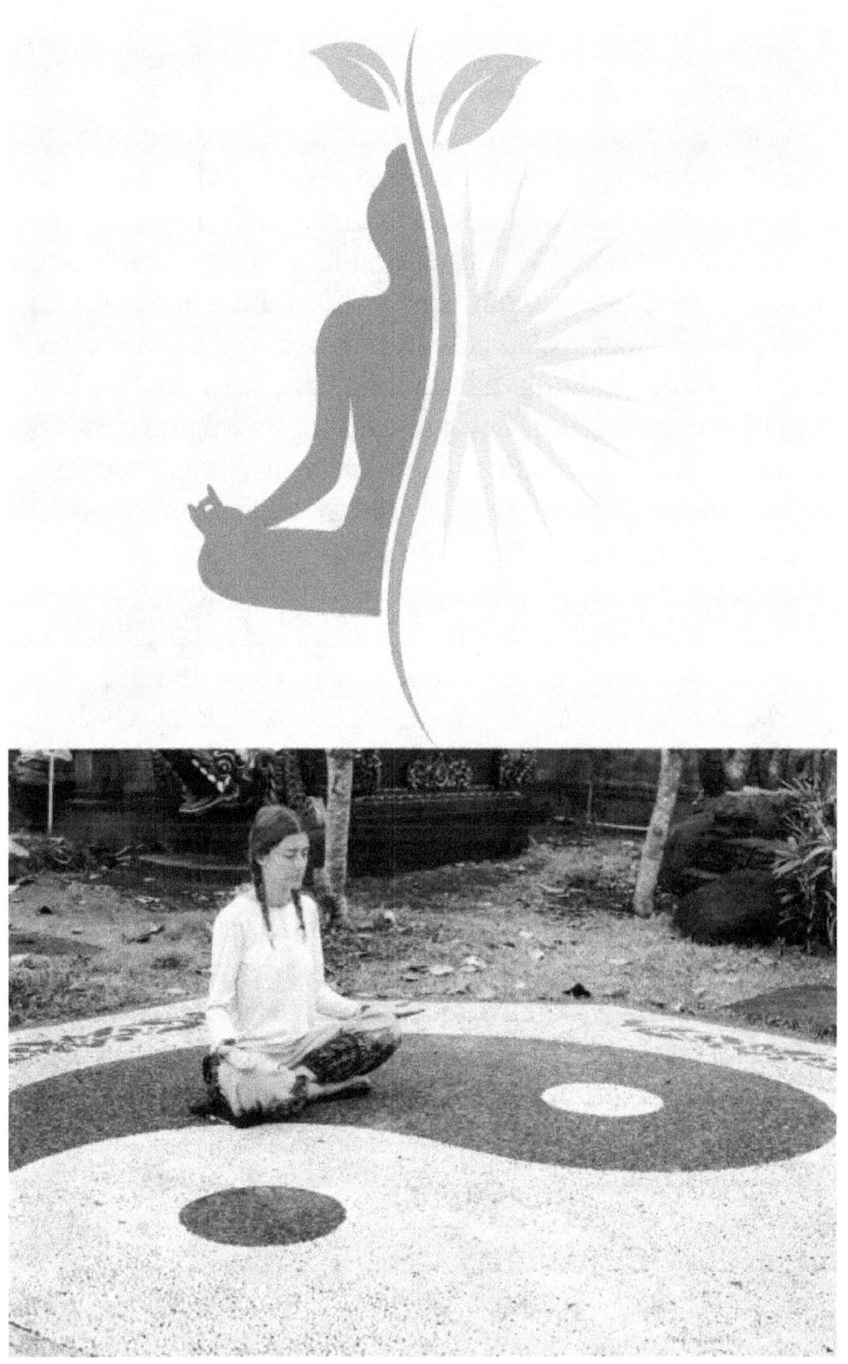

Understanding the Yin Approach to Yoga

In a world often dominated by fast-paced, high-intensity activities, the Yin approach to yoga offers a refreshing and transformative perspective. Unlike the dynamic and active Yang practices, Yin Yoga is characterized by long-held, passive postures that target the deeper connective tissues of the body, such as ligaments, joints, and fascia. Founded on the Taoist concept of balancing opposing forces, Yin and Yang, Yin Yoga embodies the principle of stillness and surrender. Central to Yin Yoga is the idea of finding ease within discomfort. As we settle into each posture, we resist the urge to force our bodies into submission, but instead, invite relaxation and let gravity gently guide us deeper. The practice encourages an attitude of acceptance, allowing sensations to arise and pass without judgment or resistance. By nurturing this state of surrender, practitioners cultivate a profound sense of patience and self-compassion that transcends the mat and spills into daily life.

The slow pace of Yin Yoga also fosters introspection and self-reflection. In the stillness of the postures, we gain insight into the workings of our minds and emotions. It becomes a meditative journey, where we observe thoughts and feelings without attachment, making space for self-discovery and growth. This profound sense of self-awareness serves as a powerful tool in cultivating inner strength and flexibility.

The Benefits of Cultivating Inner Strength and Flexibility

At first glance, the idea of cultivating "inner" strength and flexibility might seem abstract, but its effects ripple throughout our entire being. Inner strength is not about brute force or rigid determination; it is a profound reservoir of resilience, courage, and emotional fortitude that enables us to navigate life's challenges with grace. Inner strength empowers us to remain steady in the face of adversity, to bounce back from setbacks, and to maintain composure during turbulent times. As we delve deeper into Yin Yoga, we uncover the interconnectedness of body, mind, and spirit. The practice of holding postures for an extended period fosters mental endurance and the ability to embrace discomfort with equanimity. By learning to soften around discomfort instead of resisting it, we develop the capacity to face difficult emotions and situations with greater composure. This emotional flexibility is a valuable asset in building inner strength. Moreover, Yin Yoga nourishes the subtle energy systems of the body, such as the meridians in Traditional Chinese Medicine or the nadis in Ayurveda. As these energy channels are unblocked and balanced,

our life force (prana or chi) flows freely, promoting physical and emotional harmony. This revitalization not only contributes to a healthier body but also supports mental and emotional well-being, reinforcing our inner strength.

Simultaneously, cultivating flexibility goes beyond physical prowess. Yin Yoga encourages us to be open-minded, adaptable, and receptive to change. When we resist rigidity and embrace flexibility, we learn to flow with life's unfolding circumstances, embracing impermanence as a natural part of existence. This mental flexibility equips us to adapt to ever-changing situations with ease, reducing stress and promoting emotional equilibrium.

Mindfulness and Its Role in the Practice

At the heart of Yoga Yin lies the practice of mindfulness - a state of non-judgmental awareness of the present moment. Mindfulness is the thread that weaves through every aspect of Yin Yoga, guiding us into a deeper understanding of our bodies, minds, and emotions. It encourages us to be fully present, to immerse ourselves in the sensations of each posture, and to observe the fluctuations of the mind without attachment. In the context of Yin Yoga, mindfulness enhances the quality of our practice. By staying attuned to our breath, sensations, and thoughts, we cultivate a profound connection with ourselves. This heightened awareness allows us to recognize areas of tension and release them with gentleness and compassion. As we deepen our mindfulness practice, we become more receptive to the subtle messages our bodies convey, paving the way for profound physical and emotional healing.

Mindfulness also serves as an anchor during the long holds of Yin postures. When the mind wanders or discomfort arises, mindfulness guides us back to the present moment, reminding us to embrace the experience without judgment. This practice of returning to the breath and the body in the face of distraction is a metaphor for life, where we continually redirect our focus to what truly matters amid life's distractions.

Preparing the Mind and Body for Yoga Yin

Before stepping onto the mat for a Yin Yoga practice, it is essential to set the stage for a meaningful and transformative experience. Preparing the mind and body involves creating a conducive environment and nurturing the right mindset.

Create a Tranquil Space: Find a quiet and clutter-free space where you can practice without interruption. Dim the lights, light candles, or play soothing

music to create a serene atmosphere that supports relaxation and introspection.

Gather Props: Gather the necessary props to support your practice. Yin Yoga often requires props such as bolsters, blocks, and blankets to provide comfort and stability during long holds. These props enable you to relax into postures without strain, allowing the body to soften and surrender.

Set an Intention: Take a moment to set an intention for your practice. It could be as simple as cultivating patience, embracing self-compassion, or exploring a specific emotion or challenge. Let this intention guide your practice, infusing it with purpose and meaning.

Warm-Up Mindfully: Unlike Yang practices, Yin Yoga does not require a vigorous warm-up. However, a gentle warm-up sequence can prepare the body for deeper stretching. Focus on mobilizing the joints and gently stretching the muscles before moving into Yin postures.

Cultivate Patience and Let Go of Expectations: In Yin Yoga, progress is measured not by achieving advanced poses but by the depth of surrender and self-awareness. Embrace the practice with patience and curiosity, releasing any expectations of achieving certain outcomes.

Listen to Your Body: Honour the wisdom of your body. As you move into postures, listen to the signals it sends you. Avoid pushing beyond your limits and learn to differentiate between discomfort and pain. Find your edge in each posture and breathe into it with gentleness.

The foundations of Yoga Yin are built on the principles of stillness, surrender, mindfulness, and self-compassion. Understanding the Yin approach to yoga empowers us to explore the depths of inner strength and flexibility, fostering resilience and adaptability in the face of life's challenges. By cultivating mindfulness, we enrich our practice, tapping into the transformative power of the present moment. Preparing the mind and body creates a sacred space for self-exploration and growth, as we embark on a journey that transcends the boundaries of the mat, infusing every aspect of our lives with tranquillity and empowerment. As we move forward in this book, we invite you to embrace the essence of Yoga Yin and discover the profound treasures that await within.

Chapter 2
Embracing Stillness and Surrender

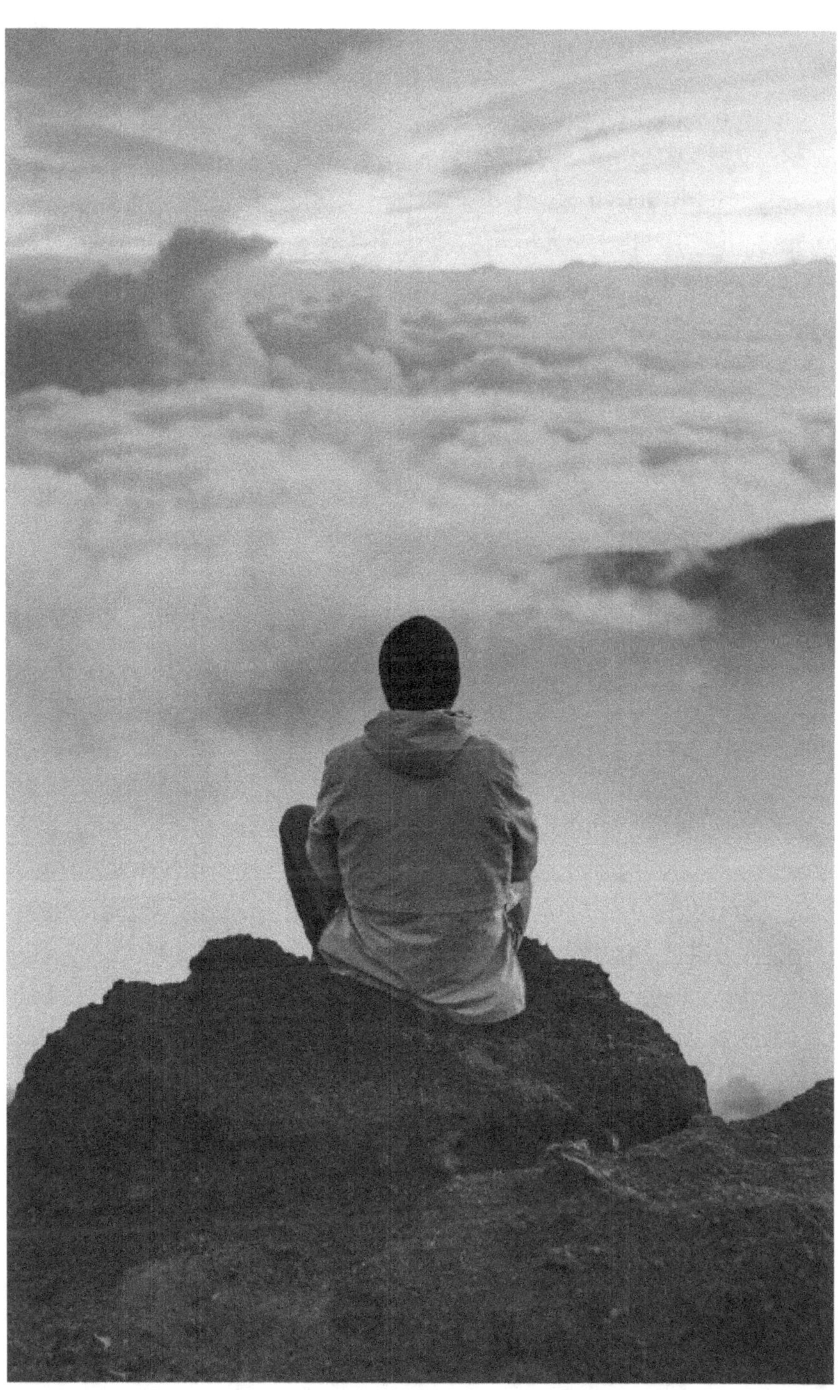

In the fast-paced world we inhabit, stillness is often undervalued and overlooked. We find ourselves constantly on the move, filling every moment with activity and distraction, leaving little room for quiet contemplation. However, in the realm of Yin Yoga, stillness is a powerful practice that invites us to let go of the need to do and achieve, and instead, embrace the art of surrender. In this chapter, we delve deep into the heart of stillness and surrender, exploring how these transformative qualities enrich our Yin Yoga practice and permeate our lives.

The Art of Surrendering in Yin Postures

In Yin Yoga, postures are typically held for an extended duration, often ranging from two to five minutes or even longer. These long holds create an opportunity to explore the art of surrender fully. As we settle into a Yin posture, we encounter sensations that challenge our desire for control and comfort. Instead of resisting or avoiding discomfort, we learn to soften and surrender, allowing gravity to guide us deeper into the posture. The practice of surrender is not synonymous with giving up or passivity. On the contrary, it is an act of profound courage and self-awareness. Surrendering in Yin postures calls for the willingness to meet the edges of discomfort with curiosity and compassion. It involves letting go of the need to control outcomes and trusting in the wisdom of our bodies. Through surrender, we release the grip of tension and resistance that accumulates in the body and mind. We become witnesses to the ebb and flow of sensations, observing without attachment or judgment. Surrendering cultivates a sense of humility and openness, acknowledging that there is much we do not know or understand. It is an invitation to meet ourselves exactly as we are, accepting our strengths, vulnerabilities, and limitations with equanimity.

Developing Patience and Resilience

Patience is a virtue often praised but seldom practised in our modern world of instant gratification. Yin Yoga offers a sanctuary for nurturing this essential quality. The prolonged holds of Yin postures challenge us to relinquish the need for quick results and to embrace the process of transformation over time. As we remain in a Yin posture, the mind may become restless, seeking release and movement. Developing patience is an invitation to befriend this restlessness, acknowledging its presence without succumbing to its demands. With time and practice, patience becomes an ally that supports us both on and off the mat.

Patience is deeply intertwined with resilience. In Yin Yoga, we confront

discomfort without seeking immediate relief. This resilience is not a hardening or toughening of the spirit but a gentle surrender to the natural rhythm of life. Just as the seasons transition and flow, our emotions and experiences ebb and flow. Resilience allows us to embrace the impermanence of life with grace, knowing that every sensation, emotion, and circumstance is transient.

Releasing Tension and Stress Through Stillness

In our hectic lives, stress and tension tend to accumulate in the body and mind, creating a perpetual state of disquiet. The practice of stillness in Yin Yoga offers a powerful antidote to this modern-day affliction. By settling into Yin postures, we create a safe space to release the accumulated tension, both physical and mental. During the long holds of Yin postures, the fascia, a connective tissue that surrounds muscles and organs, is gently stretched and stimulated. This process not only enhances flexibility but also aids in the release of tension stored in the fascia. As we breathe into the sensations that arise, we encourage the gradual melting of muscular tension, promoting a sense of deep relaxation.

Moreover, the stillness of Yin Yoga provides an opportunity to address the mental and emotional stress that we carry within. When the mind is constantly preoccupied with worries and distractions, it rarely finds the chance to unwind. In the tranquillity of stillness, we create space to observe our thoughts and feelings with non-judgmental awareness, fostering a sense of inner calm and clarity.

Breathing Techniques for Enhanced Relaxation

The breath is an essential anchor in any yoga practice, and Yin Yoga is no exception. As we hold Yin postures, the breath becomes a source of solace and relaxation, guiding us through the experience with mindfulness and ease.

Incorporating specific breathing techniques in Yin Yoga enhances relaxation and supports the body's natural healing processes. One such technique is diaphragmatic breathing, also known as belly breathing or deep breathing. This technique involves breathing deeply into the abdomen, allowing the diaphragm to expand fully. As the breath flows deeply and rhythmically, it activates the parasympathetic nervous system, which counteracts the stress response and induces a state of relaxation.

In Yin postures, we can focus on the breath to ease into the discomfort and remain present. By directing the breath to areas of tension or resistance, we facilitate the release of held emotions and stagnant energy, inviting a sense of

spaciousness and openness. Additionally, breath awareness during Yin postures helps us navigate the fine line between sensation and pain. Pain is a signal to back off from a posture, while sensation can be an opportunity to explore and soften. The breath becomes a gentle guide, revealing our edges and guiding us toward a balanced and sustainable practice.

Embracing stillness and surrender in Yin Yoga is an art form that nurtures patience, resilience, and relaxation. The long holds of Yin postures offer a sacred space to release tension, both physical and emotional, and cultivate a profound sense of self-awareness. Surrendering invites us to meet ourselves with compassion, acknowledging our vulnerabilities as part of the human experience. As we delve deeper into the practice of stillness, we discover the transformative power of patience and resilience, empowering us to navigate life's challenges with grace and equanimity. Breath becomes our ally, guiding us through the practice with mindfulness and enhanced relaxation. The art of stillness and surrender extends far beyond the mat, infusing every aspect of our lives with tranquillity, self-compassion, and serenity. In the chapters that follow, we continue to explore the essence of Yoga Yin, unveiling the profound treasures that lie within each breath, each pose, and each moment of surrender.

Chapter 3
Unleashing the Power of Breath

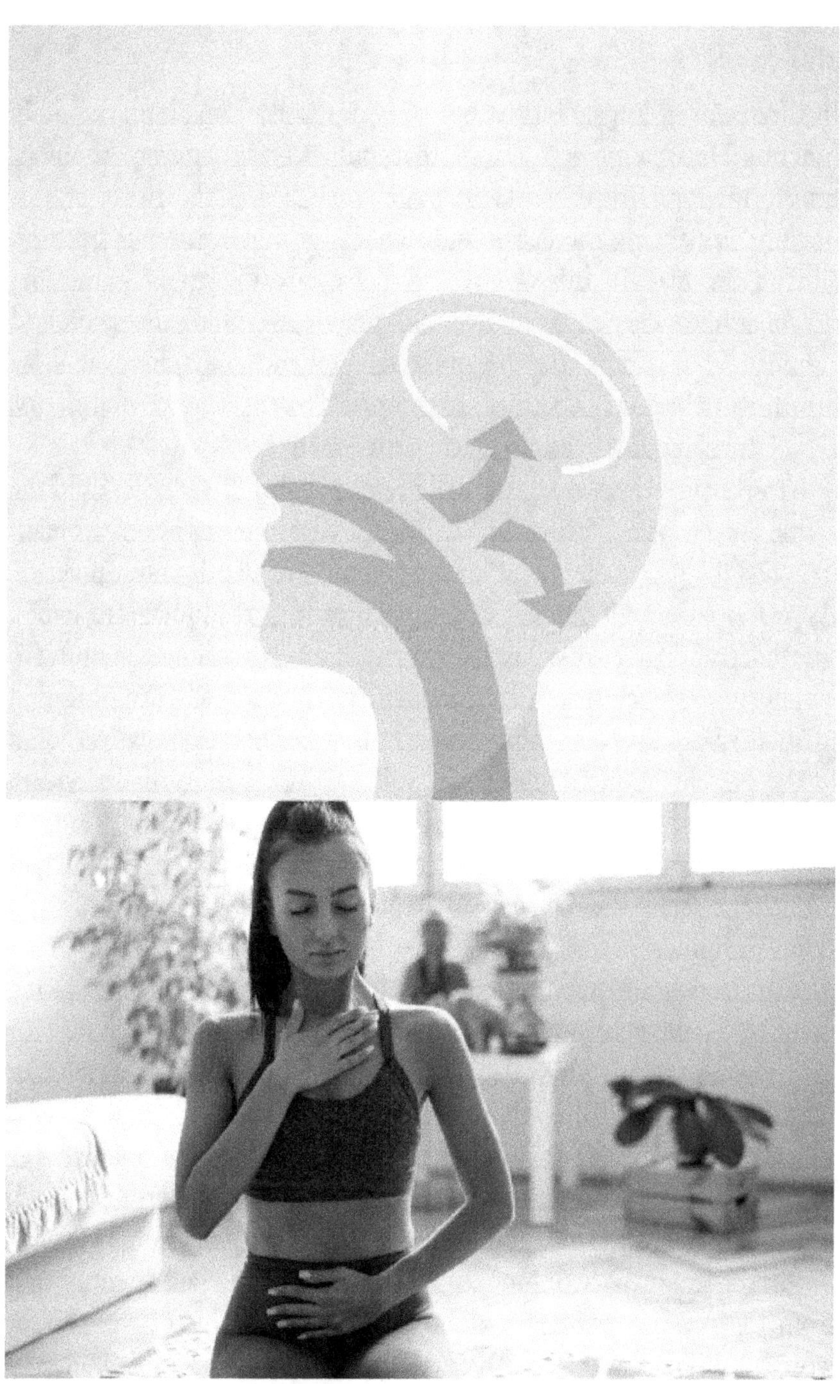

In the realm of Yoga Yin, the breath is not just an involuntary bodily function; it is a powerful tool that unlocks the gateway to inner transformation. Breath-work, or pranayama, lies at the heart of this practice, enhancing the depth and richness of our experience both on and off the mat. In this chapter, we delve into the art of harnessing the breath to deepen our Yoga Yin practice, explore the profound connection it offers to the present moment, and discover how breath-work becomes a pathway to emotional balance and mental clarity.

Harnessing the Breath to Deepen the Practice

The breath serves as an essential bridge between the physical and the subtle aspects of our being. In Yin Yoga, we learn to harness the breath to access the present moment and to enhance the depth of our practice. As we move through the gentle postures, breath-work guides us to soften, surrender, and let go of resistance. Incorporating conscious breathing in Yin postures transforms them from mere physical stretches to profound meditative experiences. The breath acts as an anchor, keeping us rooted in the present moment amidst the stillness. With each inhalation, we invite space and openness into the body, and with each exhalation, we release tension and discomfort. This rhythmic dance of breath and movement establishes a harmonious flow that nurtures the body and calms the mind.

The breath also serves as an indicator of our state of being during practice. Shallow and constricted breathing may signify physical or emotional tension, while deep and steady breaths signal a state of relaxation and ease. Through mindful observation of the breath, we gain valuable insights into our physical and emotional landscape, making way for conscious adjustments and a deeper connection with ourselves.

Connecting with the Present Moment through Pranayama

In the frantic pace of modern life, it is easy to become disconnected from the present moment, constantly lost in thoughts of the past or worries about the future. Pranayama, or breath-work, becomes a powerful vehicle to anchor ourselves firmly in the here and now. As we tune into the breath, we shift our attention from the external world to the internal landscape of sensations, thoughts, and emotions. Pranayama in Yin Yoga is not about controlling the breath but about observing it with gentle awareness. Various breathing techniques can be integrated into Yin postures, such as extended exhalations, abdominal breathing, and alternate nostril breathing. These practices infuse the

practice with mindfulness, facilitating a deepening of self-awareness. One of the simplest and most accessible pranayama practices in Yin Yoga is the 4-7-8 breath. To practice this technique, inhale deeply for a count of four, hold the breath for a count of seven, and exhale slowly for a count of eight. This breath-work technique helps to calm the nervous system and bring a sense of centeredness and tranquillity.

Through pranayama, we learn to become witnesses to the ever-changing flow of the breath, mirroring the impermanent nature of life. As we breathe consciously, we begin to embrace the present moment without resistance, cultivating a state of acceptance and contentment.

Breath-work for Emotional Balance and Mental Clarity

Our breath is intricately connected to our emotional state. Notice how the breath quickens when we feel anxious or stressed and how it deepens when we experience relaxation and joy. In Yin Yoga, we can intentionally use the breath to regulate our emotions, finding emotional balance and mental clarity. When we encounter challenges in Yin postures, such as discomfort or resistance, the breath acts as a guide to navigate through these moments with ease. By breathing consciously into areas of tension, we direct the breath to soften and release physical and emotional holding. This process allows us to approach challenges with a calm and composed mind, transforming moments of struggle into opportunities for growth and self-compassion.

Breath-work is also a powerful tool to regulate our emotional responses off the mat. By consciously slowing down the breath during moments of stress or agitation, we engage the parasympathetic nervous system, triggering the relaxation response. This practice not only helps us regain emotional equilibrium but also fosters mental clarity and sound decision-making. Through breath-work, we cultivate emotional intelligence, learning to recognize and honour our emotions without becoming overwhelmed by them. As we develop a steady and conscious relationship with the breath, we embrace the full spectrum of human emotions with equanimity, finding freedom in the space between each inhale and exhale.

The power of the breath in Yoga Yin is a gateway to deepening the practice, connecting with the present moment, and fostering emotional balance and mental clarity. By harnessing the breath, we infuse our practice with mindfulness, embracing the beauty of each moment with conscious awareness.

Breath-work allows us to navigate the stillness and surrender of Yin postures with grace and self-compassion. The breath serves as a constant anchor, guiding us back to the present moment when the mind wanders or discomfort arises. Through pranayama, we explore the intimate connection between our breath and our emotional state, enabling us to find balance and resilience in the face of life's challenges. As we integrate the power of breath into our Yin Yoga practice, we embark on a journey of profound self-discovery and transformation. Breath becomes our faithful companion, leading us to a place of inner stillness and peace, where we discover the boundless treasures that reside within each breath and each precious moment. In the chapters that follow, we continue to explore the essence of Yoga Yin, unveiling the transformative potential that awaits through the gateway of the breath.

Chapter 4
Nurturing the Body-Mind Connection

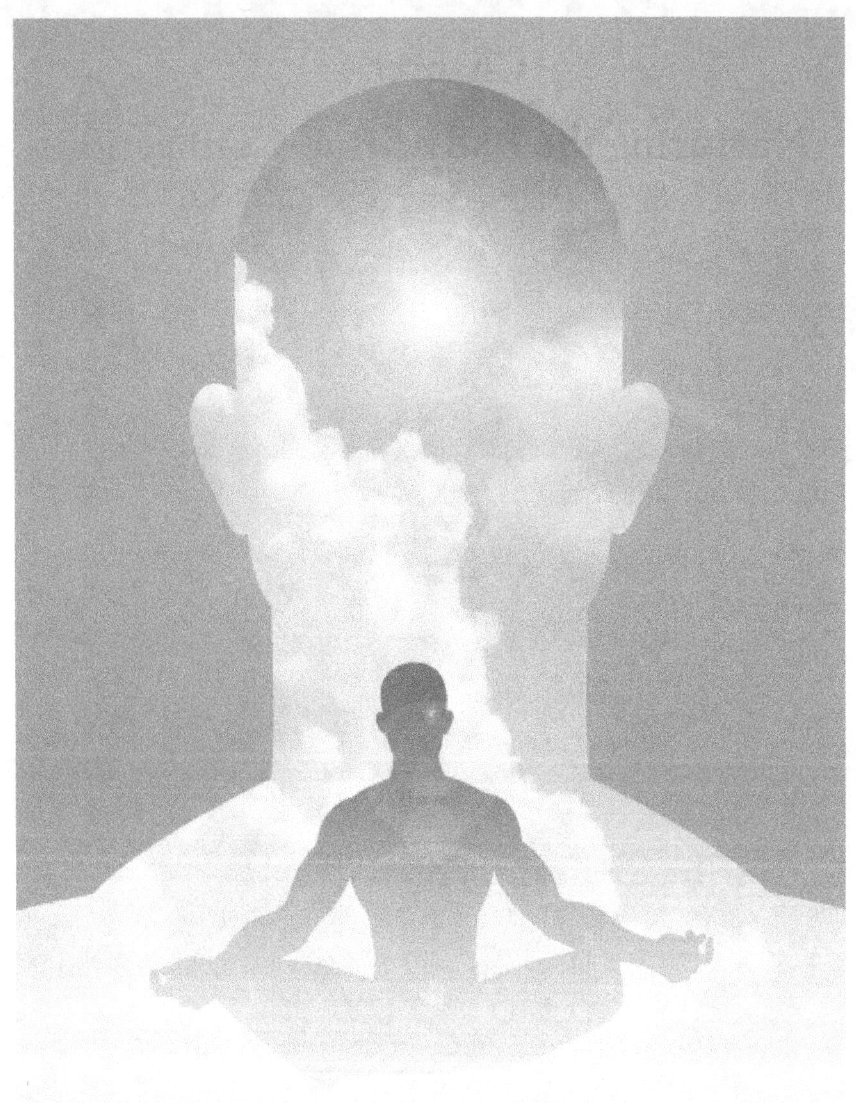

In the realm of Yoga Yin, the practice transcends the mere physicality of yoga asanas. It delves deep into the essence of the mind-body connection, revealing the profound interplay between our physical sensations and mental states. This chapter explores how Yoga Yin invites us to explore and nurture this intimate connection, cultivating self-awareness, mindfulness, and the art of listening to the body's wisdom and intuition.

Exploring the Mind-Body Connection in Yoga Yin

The mind-body connection is the intricate communication network that links our thoughts, emotions, and physical sensations. In the context of Yoga Yin, this connection becomes palpable as we move through the gentle postures and embrace the stillness. Unlike more dynamic practices, Yin Yoga offers us the time and space to witness and explore the interplay between our body and mind. As we settle into Yin postures, we may encounter physical sensations that evoke emotional responses. For example, tight hips might trigger feelings of resistance or vulnerability. Conversely, a deep sense of release in the shoulders might lead to emotional ease and openness. In Yoga Yin, we become attentive observers of these connections, noticing how our mental states influence our physical sensations and vice versa.

The exploration of the mind-body connection becomes a journey of self-discovery, revealing the deeply ingrained patterns and habits that shape our experiences on and off the mat. Through this awareness, we gain insight into the subtle ways our emotions manifest in the body and how our physical experiences affect our mental landscape.

Cultivating Self-Awareness and Mindfulness

Self-awareness is the foundation upon which the practice of Yoga Yin is built. It is the art of turning inward and observing our thoughts, emotions, and bodily sensations without judgment. Through self-awareness, we become intimate witnesses of the present moment, acknowledging our experiences with compassionate curiosity. In Yin postures, self-awareness guides us to remain present with the breath and sensations. We notice the ever-changing flow of the breath, the subtle shifts in the body, and the arising and passing of thoughts and emotions. This practice of mindfulness grounds us in the present moment, liberating us from the grip of past regrets and future anxieties.

Mindfulness in Yoga Yin extends beyond the mat, permeating our daily lives

with clarity and presence. By bringing mindful awareness to our actions and interactions, we respond to life's challenges with intention and wisdom, rather than reacting impulsively.

Listening to the Body's Wisdom and Intuition

The body is a repository of innate wisdom and intuition that speaks to us in whispers. In the stillness of Yin Yoga, we hone our ability to listen attentively to these gentle messages. As we hold Yin postures, the body communicates its needs, desires, and boundaries through physical sensations. The art of listening to the body requires us to approach the practice with sensitivity and non-judgmental awareness. We learn to distinguish between sensations that signal healthy stretching and those that indicate discomfort or strain. By honouring the body's wisdom, we avoid pushing ourselves beyond our limits, cultivating a safe and sustainable practice. Beyond the physical level, the body also communicates through emotional responses. For example, we may encounter emotional releases during Yin postures, such as tears or feelings of vulnerability. Instead of suppressing these experiences, we allow them to unfold with compassion, acknowledging that emotional healing is an integral part of our practice. As we deepen our practice of listening to the body's wisdom, we develop a profound trust in our intuition. The body's messages become a reliable guide, steering us toward choices and actions that align with our authentic selves. This intuitive connection empowers us to make decisions that resonate with our deepest values and aspirations.

Nurturing the body-mind connection in Yoga Yin is a transformative journey of self-awareness, mindfulness, and intuitive wisdom. Through the practice, we explore the intricate interplay between physical sensations, emotions, and mental states, unveiling the patterns that shape our experiences. Cultivating self-awareness and mindfulness anchors us in the present moment, freeing us from the chains of past regrets and future anxieties. The practice of self-awareness extends beyond the mat, infusing our daily lives with clarity and intention. By listening attentively to the body's wisdom and intuition, we honour our physical and emotional boundaries, fostering a safe and nurturing practice. The body becomes our trusted guide, steering us toward choices that align with our true selves. Through the profound exploration of the body-mind connection in Yoga Yin, we unveil the vast landscape of self-discovery and self-empowerment. The practice becomes a transformative journey, unveiling the boundless treasures that reside within each breath, each sensation, and each moment of stillness.

Chapter 5
Cultivating Inner Strength

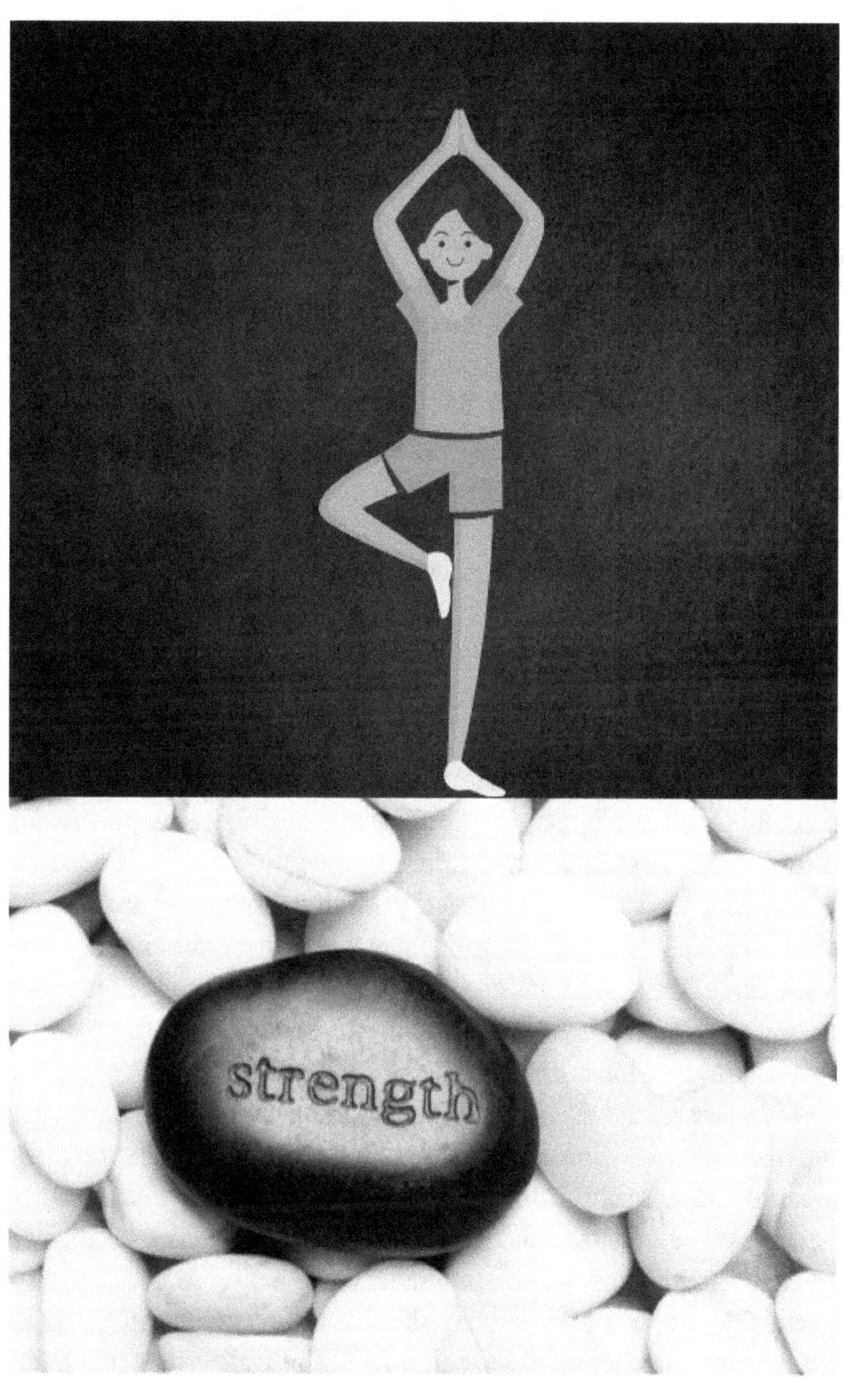

In the gentle embrace of Yoga Yin, we discover that inner strength is not solely a product of physical prowess or external achievements; it is a profound reservoir of resilience and empowerment that lies within each of us. This chapter explores how Yoga Yin becomes a catalyst for cultivating mental resilience, tapping into our inner resources and confidence, and empowering us to overcome challenges both on and off the mat.

Building Mental Resilience through the Practice

Mental resilience is the ability to bounce back from setbacks, adapt to change, and navigate life's challenges with composure and fortitude. In Yoga Yin, we build mental resilience by confronting moments of discomfort and surrendering to the present moment with equanimity. The long holds of Yin postures present us with a unique opportunity to explore our mental responses to physical sensations. As we encounter discomfort, resistance, or impatience, we practice mental resilience by remaining present and observing these reactions without judgment. We learn to soften around discomfort, finding ease within the challenge, and embracing the impermanence of each sensation. The practice of mental resilience extends beyond the mat and into our daily lives. As we develop the capacity to face physical discomfort with grace, we transfer this resilience to face emotional and mental challenges with similar poise. Yoga Yin becomes a training ground for cultivating a resilient mind that navigates the ever-changing tides of life with courage and ease.

Tapping into Inner Resources and Confidence

Yoga Yin provides a sanctuary for accessing our inner resources and fostering self-confidence. Each time we settle into a Yin posture, we tap into our reservoir of strength and stillness, drawing upon our inner reserves to sustain us through the long holds. With each breath, we cultivate a sense of inner steadiness that transcends the external fluctuations of life. As we embrace the art of surrender in Yin postures, we cultivate trust in our bodies and minds. This trust is the foundation of self-confidence, the unwavering belief in our abilities and the innate wisdom of our intuition. With each Yin practice, we deepen our connection with our inner selves, and in doing so, we cultivate a profound sense of self-assurance. The empowerment gained through Yoga Yin becomes a guiding force that influences our actions and choices in daily life. As we navigate challenges off the mat, we draw upon this inner strength and confidence to make decisions aligned with our values and aspirations. We no longer seek validation from external sources but find reassurance from the

unwavering wellspring of strength within.

Overcoming Challenges on and off the Mat

Yoga Yin becomes a training ground for overcoming challenges both physical and emotional. The practice invites us to meet moments of discomfort with self-compassion, acknowledging that growth often springs from the most challenging experiences. On the mat, we confront physical resistance and mental restlessness, learning to breathe through moments of discomfort and resistance. We embrace the process of transformation, trusting that with time and patience, even the most challenging postures become accessible. Off the mat, the mental resilience and inner strength we cultivate in Yoga Yin empower us to face life's adversities with grace. We approach challenges with a mindset of curiosity and openness, knowing that each obstacle carries the potential for growth and self-discovery. Yoga Yin becomes a sanctuary where we learn not to shy away from challenges but to embrace them as opportunities for self-realization. The practice fosters a spirit of resilience and tenacity, empowering us to confront life's uncertainties with a sense of empowerment and groundedness.

Cultivating inner strength in Yoga Yin is a transformative journey of mental resilience, tapping into our inner resources and confidence, and empowering us to overcome challenges both on and off the mat. Through the practice of mental resilience, we learn to soften around discomfort and embrace the impermanence of each moment. This resilience extends beyond the mat, empowering us to navigate life's challenges with courage and ease. In Yoga Yin, we discover a reservoir of inner strength and stillness that sustains us through the long holds of postures and in the face of life's uncertainties. Tapping into our inner resources, we foster self-confidence and trust in our abilities, empowering us to make decisions aligned with our authentic selves. Yoga Yin becomes a training ground for facing challenges with grace and curiosity, cultivating a spirit of resilience that permeates our lives.

Chapter 6
Enhancing Flexibility and Mobility

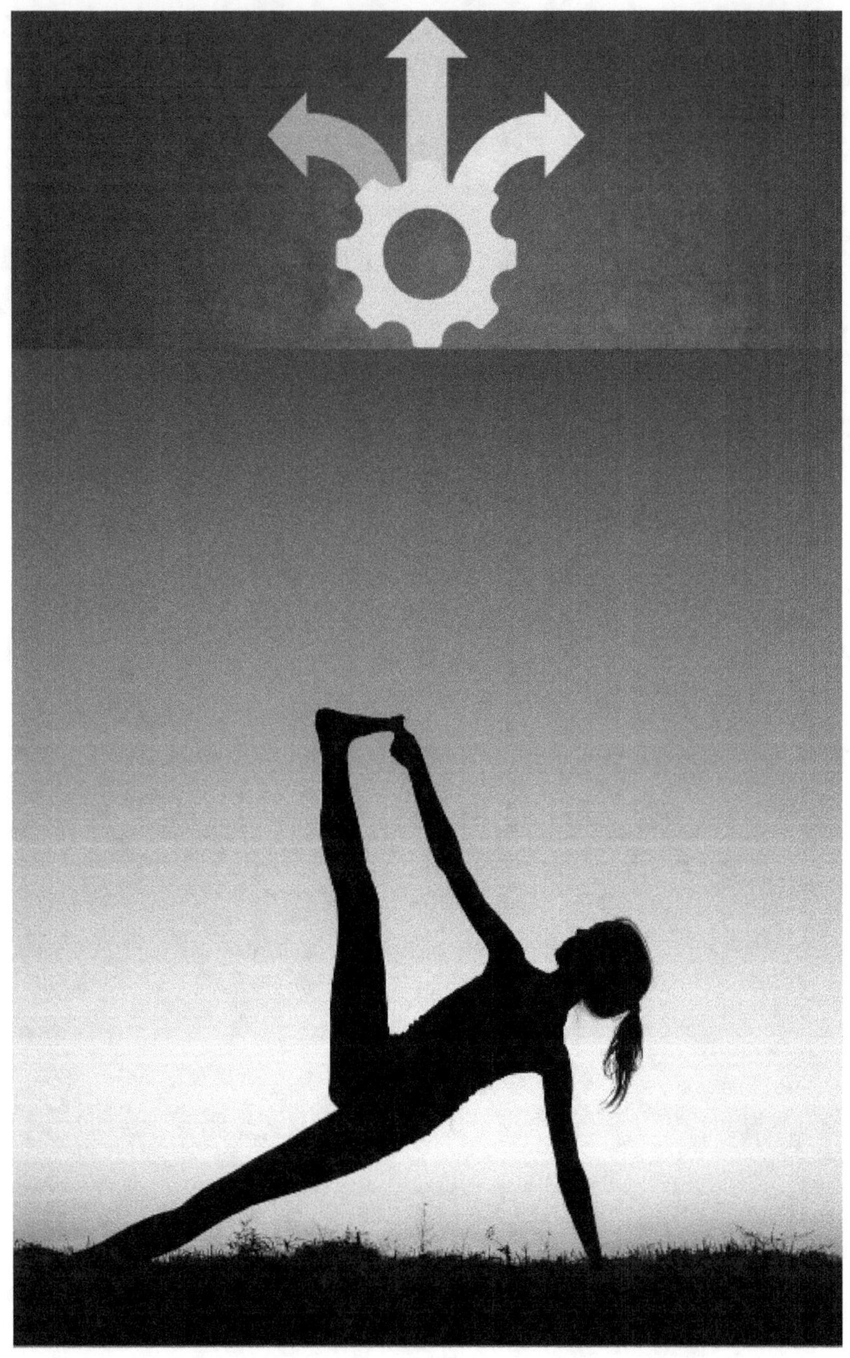

In the journey of Yoga Yin, flexibility and mobility take on a new dimension beyond the physical realm. Instead of striving for extreme contortions, Yoga Yin invites us to explore flexibility as an approach to embracing change and adapting with ease. This chapter delves into the art of enhancing flexibility and mobility in a mindful and nurturing way, working with the body's natural range of motion, harnessing the power of Yin postures to improve flexibility, and honouring our individual progress and limitations.

Working with the Body's Natural Range of Motion

Flexibility and mobility in Yoga Yin are not about forcing the body into unnatural shapes or pushing beyond its limits. Instead, we work with the body's natural range of motion, respecting its unique anatomy and physiology. The practice becomes a gentle inquiry into our body's capabilities, observing the sensations and reactions with compassion. Each individual's body is unique, and what might be accessible for one person may be challenging for another. Yoga Yin becomes an exploration of the body's innate wisdom, understanding that the natural range of motion may change from day to day. Some days, we may find ourselves more open and flexible, while other days, the body might feel more resistant. Embracing this natural ebb and flow of our physicality is an integral part of the practice. In Yoga Yin, we learn to soften around the edges of our range of motion, avoiding force or strain. Instead of pushing the body into a posture, we allow the breath to guide us gently deeper, honouring the body's signals to ease off if we encounter discomfort. This approach to flexibility nurtures a sense of self-awareness, as we learn to distinguish between healthy stretching and pain.

The Role of Yin Postures in Improving Flexibility

Yin postures play a unique role in improving flexibility and mobility. Unlike dynamic practices that focus on muscle engagement and movement, Yin Yoga targets the deeper connective tissues, such as ligaments, joints, and fascia. By holding postures for an extended duration, we gently stress these tissues, encouraging them to release and lengthen over time. In Yin postures, we settle into the stillness and surrender, allowing gravity to guide us deeper into the stretch. This passive approach to stretching is both nurturing and transformative, as we learn to trust the process of release and change.

The practice of Yin postures also involves a degree of compression, gently stimulating the joints and nourishing the synovial fluid that lubricates them. This process enhances joint health and supports mobility, allowing for greater ease of movement both on and off the mat. Moreover, Yin postures offer a space for emotional release, as we store emotions and tension in the physical body. As we soften and surrender in the postures, we may encounter emotional sensations and memories arising. By allowing these experiences to surface with non-judgmental awareness, we create space for emotional healing, contributing to a more open and receptive body.

Step-by-step guidance to create a nurturing and transformative experience on the mat:

Find a Quiet Space: Choose a peaceful and quiet space for your practice. Create an environment that allows you to immerse yourself in stillness and surrender without distractions.

Gather Props: Gather any props you might need, such as bolsters, blankets, or blocks, to support your body in the postures. Props help you maintain comfort and relaxation during the longer holds.

Set an Intention: Begin your practice by setting an intention. It could be a word, phrase, or quality you wish to cultivate during the practice, such as "peace," "release," or "self-compassion."

Warm-Up: Before diving into Yin postures, spend a few minutes warming up your body with gentle movements and stretches. Focus on the areas you intend to target during your practice.

Choose Your Postures: Select the Yin postures you want to explore during your practice. Listen to your body and choose poses that resonate with your needs and intentions for the day.

Mindful Entry and Exit: As you move into and out of each posture, do so mindfully and with ease. Avoid quick or forceful movements, allowing your body to settle into each position gradually.

Hold the Postures: Yin Yoga involves holding postures for an extended duration, typically 3-5 minutes. As you settle into each pose, find a comfortable edge where you feel a gentle stretch and sensation, but not pain.

Use Props: Utilize props to support your body in the postures. Bolsters, blankets, and blocks can be placed strategically to ease tension and create a

sense of relaxation.

Breathe and Observe: Once in the posture, focus on your breath and observe the sensations in your body. Allow your breath to flow naturally, and maintain a sense of curiosity and non-judgmental awareness.

Surrender and Release: During the long holds, practice surrendering and releasing tension. Let go of the need to control or change anything. Instead, embrace the present moment with openness and acceptance.

In the practice of Yin Yoga, the following poses are commonly explored. Remember that each individual's body is unique, and it's essential to listen to your body and modify the poses as needed to suit your needs and limitations. Hold each posture for 3-5 minutes, allowing yourself to settle into stillness and surrender with mindful awareness.

Butterfly Pose (Baddha Konasana):

- Sit on the floor with the soles of your feet together, allowing your knees to drop out to the sides.
- Gently fold forward, maintaining a straight spine, and rest

your forehead on a prop or the floor.

Dragon Pose (Dragonfly or Straddle Pose):

- Sit with your legs extended wide apart.
- Slowly hinge from your hips and fold forward, reaching your hands towards your feet or placing props in front of you for support.

Caterpillar Pose (Paschimottanasana):

- Sit with your legs extended straight in front of you.
- Hinge from your hips and fold forward, aiming to reach for your feet or use props to support your hands.

Sphinx Pose:

- Lie on your belly with your forearms on the floor and elbows under your shoulders.

- Lift your chest off the ground, keeping your hips and legs relaxed.

Seal Pose:

- From Sphinx Pose, straighten your arms, lifting your chest higher off the ground.
- Keep your hips and legs relaxed, engaging your lower back muscles to lift your torso.

Child's Pose (Balasana):

- Kneel on the floor with your big toes together and knees apart.

- Fold forward, stretching your arms in front of you and resting your forehead on the floor or a prop.

Reclining Butterfly Pose (Supta Baddha Konasana):

- Lie on your back with the soles of your feet together and knees falling out to the sides.
- Allow your arms to rest by your sides or place them on your belly and chest.

Square Pose (Fire Log or Double Pigeon):

- Sit with one leg stacked on top of the other, forming a square shape with your legs.
- If your hips allow, fold forward from your hips, maintaining a straight spine.

Shoelace Pose:

- Sit with your legs crossed, stacking one knee on top of the other.
- Fold forward, keeping your spine straight and reaching your hands towards your feet.

Supported Fish Pose (Matsyasana):

- Place a bolster or a few stacked pillows on the floor.
- Lie back on the bolster, allowing your head and shoulders to be supported while your heart center opens.

Remember, Yin Yoga is a practice of stillness and surrender. As you settle into each pose, breathe deeply and observe any sensations or emotions that arise with gentle curiosity and acceptance. Allow the practice to be a space for self-inquiry, self-compassion, and profound inner transformation.

Honouring Our Individual Progress and Limitations

The journey of enhancing flexibility and mobility in Yoga Yin is not about achieving textbook-perfect poses or comparing ourselves to others. Instead, it is an invitation to embrace our individual progress and limitations with self-compassion. In a world that often glorifies extreme flexibility, Yoga Yin becomes a refuge where we redefine success as the capacity to meet ourselves exactly where we are. We honour our bodies for their unique strengths and limitations, understanding that our physicality is an ever-evolving landscape.

Throughout the practice, we learn to listen to the body's signals and respond with kindness. We recognize that our bodies may have areas of tightness and restriction, and these become opportunities for growth rather than barriers to overcome. As we cultivate self-compassion, we also foster a sense of non-attachment to outcomes. Flexibility in Yoga Yin is not about achieving specific shapes but about finding fluidity and adaptability in the face of change. We approach the practice with a mindset of curiosity and openness, allowing ourselves to be present with whatever arises.

Enhancing flexibility and mobility in Yoga Yin is a transformative journey that goes beyond physical stretching. We work with the body's natural range of motion, embracing the ebb and flow of our physicality with self-awareness and compassion. The practice of Yin postures becomes a nurturing process of encouraging release and change, supporting joint health and emotional healing.

In the sanctuary of Yoga Yin, we redefine success as the willingness to meet ourselves exactly where we are, honouring our individual progress and limitations. The journey of flexibility becomes a journey of self-acceptance and non-attachment to outcomes, embracing change and adaptability with grace.

Chapter 7
Integrating Yin and Yang: A Holistic Approach

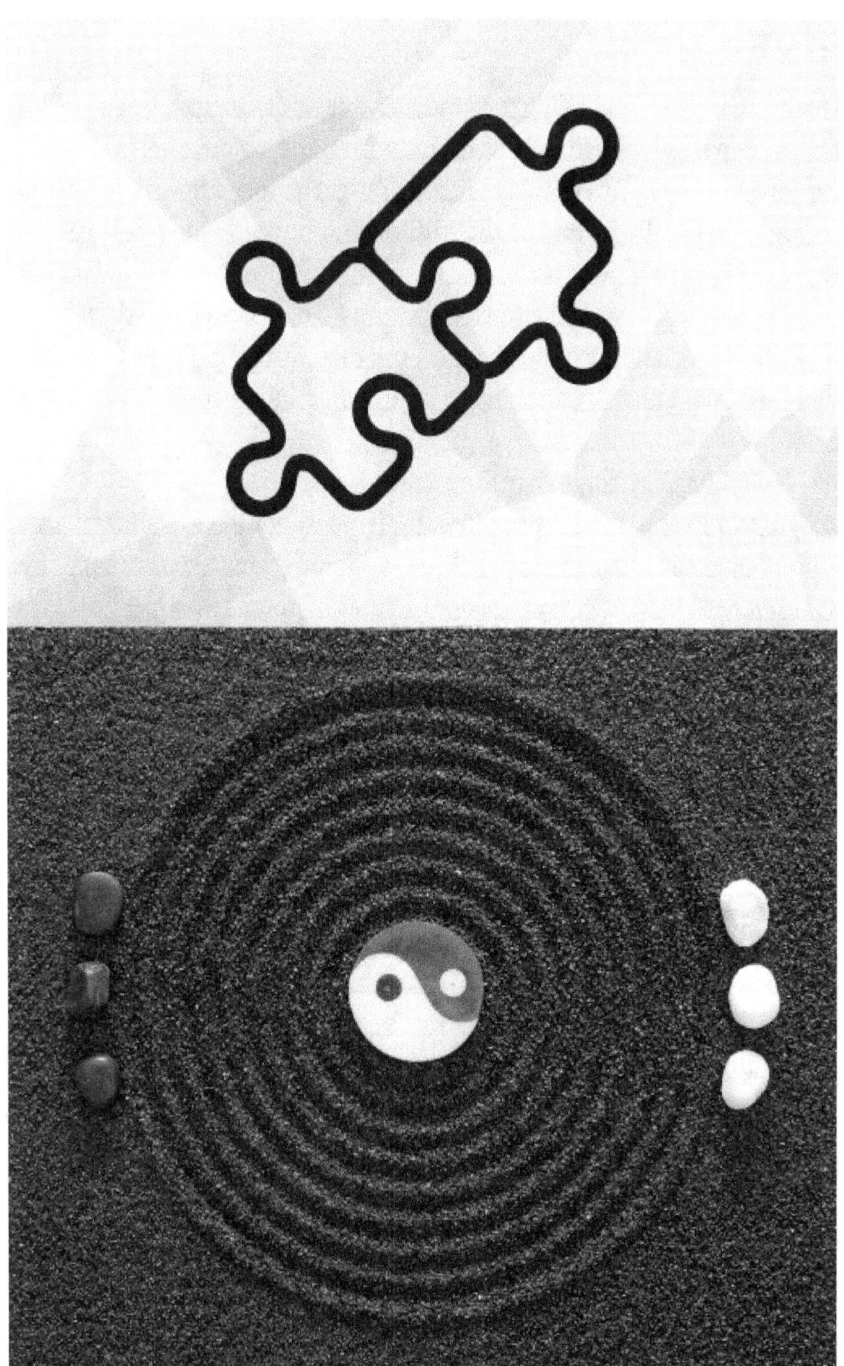

In the world of Yoga Yin, the practice does not exist in isolation but rather as part of a harmonious dance with Yang practices. This chapter explores the art of integrating Yin and Yang, creating a holistic approach to yoga and life. By balancing the stillness and surrender of Yin Yoga with the dynamism of Yang practices, we cultivate harmony and balance in our physical, mental, and emotional realms. The chapter also delves into how this integration extends beyond the mat, infusing mindfulness into daily routines and fostering a sense of presence and purpose in all aspects of life.

Balancing Yin Yoga with Yang Practices

Yoga Yin and Yang represent complementary forces in the universe, embodying the qualities of stillness and movement, receptivity and assertiveness, surrender and action. Integrating these two aspects of yoga into our practice nurtures a profound sense of equilibrium and wholeness. Yin Yoga, with its long holds and passive stretches, nourishes the deeper connective tissues and promotes relaxation. It provides a sanctuary for self-reflection, inviting us to soften and surrender to the present moment. The practice of Yin encourages introspection and self-awareness, supporting emotional healing and inner transformation. On the other hand, Yang practices, such as Vinyasa, Ashtanga, or Hatha Yoga, emphasize dynamic movements, muscular engagement, and cardiovascular exercise. These practices build strength, endurance, and focus. They stimulate the circulatory system, promoting detoxification and vitality. By combining Yin and Yang practices, we cultivate a holistic approach to yoga that honours the complexity of our being. We learn to flow with the rhythm of life, knowing when to embrace stillness and when to engage in action. The integration of Yin and Yang brings balance to our physical body, mental state, and emotional well-being.

Creating Harmony in Life through Balance

The integration of Yin and Yang extends beyond the mat, infusing our daily lives with a sense of harmony and balance. In the modern world, we often find ourselves caught in the hustle and bustle of constant activity, neglecting the need for rest and rejuvenation. The practice of Yin and Yang invites us to reclaim a sense of balance in our lives. Creating harmony through balance involves honouring the need for both rest and action. It means setting aside time for self-care, nourishing the body with healthy food, and finding moments of stillness amidst the chaos. It also means engaging in activities that bring joy and fulfilment, fostering creativity and connection with others.

Finding balance also involves being discerning about how we allocate our time and energy. It means learning to say no to activities and commitments that drain us, and yes to those that align with our values and aspirations. Through the practice of Yin and Yang, we cultivate resilience and adaptability, knowing that life's challenges are opportunities for growth and self-discovery. This holistic approach allows us to navigate life's uncertainties with grace and equanimity.

Incorporating Mindfulness into Daily Routines

Mindfulness is the thread that weaves through the fabric of Yoga Yin and Yang, infusing our practice with presence and purpose. Mindfulness is not confined to formal meditation but can be integrated into our daily routines, transforming ordinary tasks into sacred rituals of awareness. As we move through the Yin and Yang practices, we invite mindfulness to be our constant companion. Mindful movement in Yang practices allows us to stay present with each breath and each posture, cultivating a meditative flow. In Yin postures, mindfulness guides us to observe physical sensations and emotional responses with non-judgmental awareness. Beyond the mat, mindfulness becomes a way of living. We bring mindful awareness to daily activities, such as eating, walking, and interacting with others. By being fully present in each moment, we release the grip of past regrets and future anxieties, finding peace in the simplicity of the present. Mindfulness also nurtures our connection with ourselves and others. It fosters deep listening and empathy, enhancing our relationships and communication. By being fully present with others, we acknowledge their unique experiences and create a space for genuine connection.

Integrating Yin and Yang in a holistic approach to yoga and life cultivates harmony and balance in our physical, mental, and emotional realms. The dance between stillness and movement, receptivity and assertiveness, surrender and action, empowers us to flow with the rhythm of life. In the sanctuary of Yin and Yang, we find balance in our daily lives, honouring the need for rest and rejuvenation alongside dynamic engagement and action. By being discerning about how we allocate our time and energy, we create space for self-care and meaningful pursuits. Mindfulness becomes the heart of this holistic approach, infusing each moment with presence and purpose. Through mindfulness, we navigate the challenges and uncertainties of life with grace and equanimity, finding peace in the richness of the present.

Chapter 8
The Journey Within: Meditation and Yoga
Yin

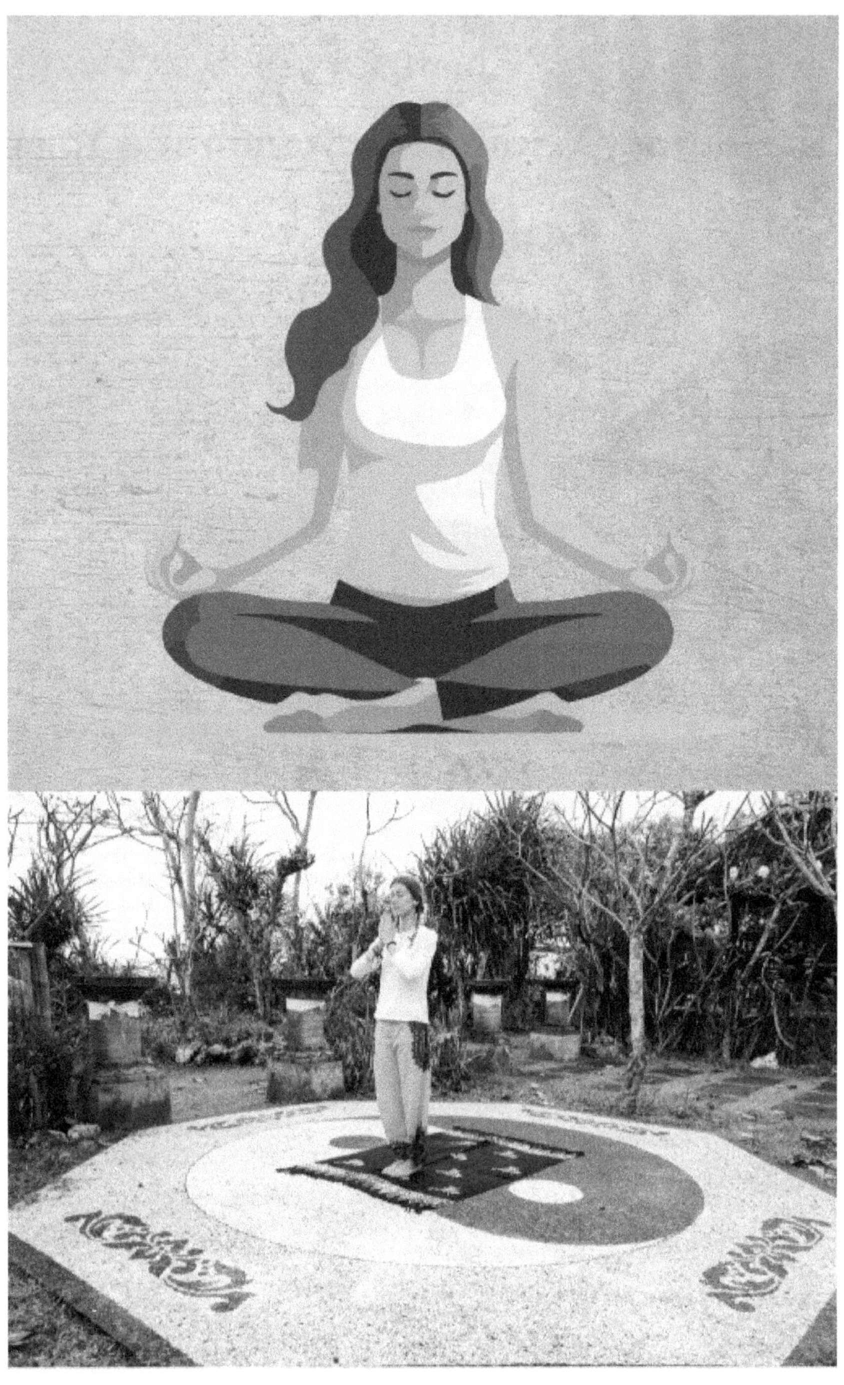

In the depths of Yoga Yin, the journey takes a profound turn as we delve into the realm of meditation and mindfulness. This chapter explores the integration of meditation with Yoga Yin, unlocking the transformative power of stillness and self-inquiry. We embark on an inner exploration of the mind and heart, using meditation as a gateway to uncover the hidden treasures within. Through the practice of Yoga Yin, we learn to harness the power of stillness for self-discovery, healing, and personal growth.

Integrating Meditation and Mindfulness with Yoga Yin

Meditation and mindfulness are natural companions to the practice of Yoga Yin, complementing each other in their pursuit of inner awareness and presence. While Yoga Yin offers a gentle approach to physical postures and relaxation, meditation takes us deeper into the subtler layers of the mind and heart. Mindfulness in Yoga Yin involves being fully present with each breath, each sensation, and each moment of surrender. By bringing focused awareness to the physical body and the breath, we cultivate a sense of mindfulness that keeps us rooted in the present moment. Integrating meditation with Yoga Yin extends this presence beyond the body and breath, guiding us to explore the inner landscape of thoughts, emotions, and mental patterns. The stillness of meditation provides a fertile ground for self-inquiry, allowing us to observe our thoughts and feelings with non-judgmental awareness. Meditation and mindfulness also become essential tools for navigating the challenges and discomfort that may arise during Yin postures. By staying present and mindful, we avoid getting entangled in thoughts of resistance or avoidance, and instead, we embrace the experience with equanimity and curiosity.

The Practice of Meditation

Find a Comfortable Seat: Sit in a comfortable cross-legged position or on a meditation cushion or chair. Ensure that your spine is straight, allowing for easy flow of breath and energy.

Relax and Ground: Take a few moments to relax your body and ground yourself. Feel the support of the earth beneath you, and let go of any tension in your muscles.

Settle Your Mind: Begin your meditation by settling your mind. You can use the breath as an anchor, focusing on the sensation of the breath entering and leaving your body.

Cultivate Stillness: Allow your body and mind to settle into stillness. If thoughts arise, simply acknowledge them without getting attached or carried away. Bring your attention back to the breath.

Explore Different Techniques: There are various meditation techniques you can explore, such as loving-kindness meditation, body scan, or mantra repetition. Find the practice that resonates with you and offers the most benefit.

Embrace the Present Moment: The essence of meditation lies in embracing the present moment fully. Cultivate a sense of presence and awareness, immersing yourself in the richness of each breath and sensation.

Practice Non-Attachment: Meditation is not about achieving a specific state or outcome. Practice non-attachment to any particular experience and embrace whatever arises with an open heart.

Set a Timer: If you are new to meditation, start with shorter sessions and gradually increase the duration as you become more comfortable. Set a timer to signal the end of your meditation practice.

End with Gratitude: As you conclude your meditation, take a moment to express gratitude for the practice and for yourself. Acknowledge the effort and commitment you put into nurturing your inner well-being.

Carry Mindfulness into Daily Life: The true essence of meditation lies in integrating mindfulness into your daily life. Carry the awareness and presence you cultivate during meditation into your interactions, tasks, and experiences throughout the day.

The practice of Yin Yoga and meditation offers a profound and transformative journey into the depths of inner strength, flexibility, and mindfulness. As you embark on this path, remember that it is a journey of exploration, self-discovery, and growth. Be patient with yourself, and let go of any expectations or judgments. Embrace each moment with a sense of curiosity and openness. Allow the practice to unfold naturally, guiding you toward a deeper connection with your body, mind, and heart. May the fusion of Yin Yoga and meditation become a source of nourishment, healing, and self-empowerment. May it become a sanctuary where you can immerse yourself in the beauty of stillness and surrender, cultivating a profound sense of inner peace and well-being.

Exploring the Inner Landscape through Meditation

In Yoga Yin, we embark on an inner journey of self-discovery through meditation. As we settle into stillness, we become observers of our inner world, witnessing the ebb and flow of thoughts, emotions, and sensations. Meditation allows us to explore the habitual patterns of the mind, revealing the ways in which our thoughts shape our experiences. By cultivating a sense of detachment, we learn not to identify with our thoughts and emotions, recognizing them as passing clouds in the vast sky of consciousness. In this inner exploration, we may encounter aspects of ourselves that we have avoided or suppressed. Meditation becomes a sanctuary for embracing the entirety of our being, with all its light and shadow. By offering compassionate attention to every aspect of ourselves, we foster a sense of self-acceptance and wholeness. Beyond the surface layers of the mind, meditation takes us to the depths of the heart. We open ourselves to vulnerability and rawness, discovering the wellsprings of compassion and love that reside within. In the stillness, we find an inner sanctuary where we can connect with our true essence.

Harnessing Stillness for Self-Discovery and Growth

The stillness of Yoga Yin becomes a potent medium for self-discovery and personal growth. In a world that often glorifies busyness and productivity, the practice of stillness becomes a rebellion of self-care and introspection. By immersing ourselves in stillness, we create space to listen to the whispers of the soul. The external noise fades, and we attune ourselves to the inner guidance that speaks to us with clarity and wisdom. In this space of silence, we tap into the well of intuition and creativity that lies within. As we harness the power of stillness, we gain insights into the patterns that govern our lives. We observe the ways in which we react to challenges, how we respond to stress, and what brings us joy and fulfilment. With this awareness, we can make conscious choices that align with our authentic selves. The practice of stillness in Yoga Yin also becomes a portal for emotional healing and release. As we surrender to the present moment, we may encounter emotions that have been buried or suppressed. By offering them compassionate attention, we create space for healing and transformation.

The integration of meditation and mindfulness with Yoga Yin opens a portal to the inner landscape, allowing us to explore the depths of our mind and heart. By being fully present with each moment, we cultivate a sense of mindfulness that keeps us rooted in the present.

Through meditation, we embark on a journey of self-discovery, observing our thoughts, emotions, and mental patterns with non-judgmental awareness. Meditation becomes a sanctuary for embracing our authentic selves, with all our light and shadow. The stillness of Yoga Yin becomes a fertile ground for personal growth and transformation. By immersing ourselves in the practice of stillness, we tap into our inner wisdom and intuition, gaining insights into the patterns that govern our lives.

Chapter 9
Embracing Transformation

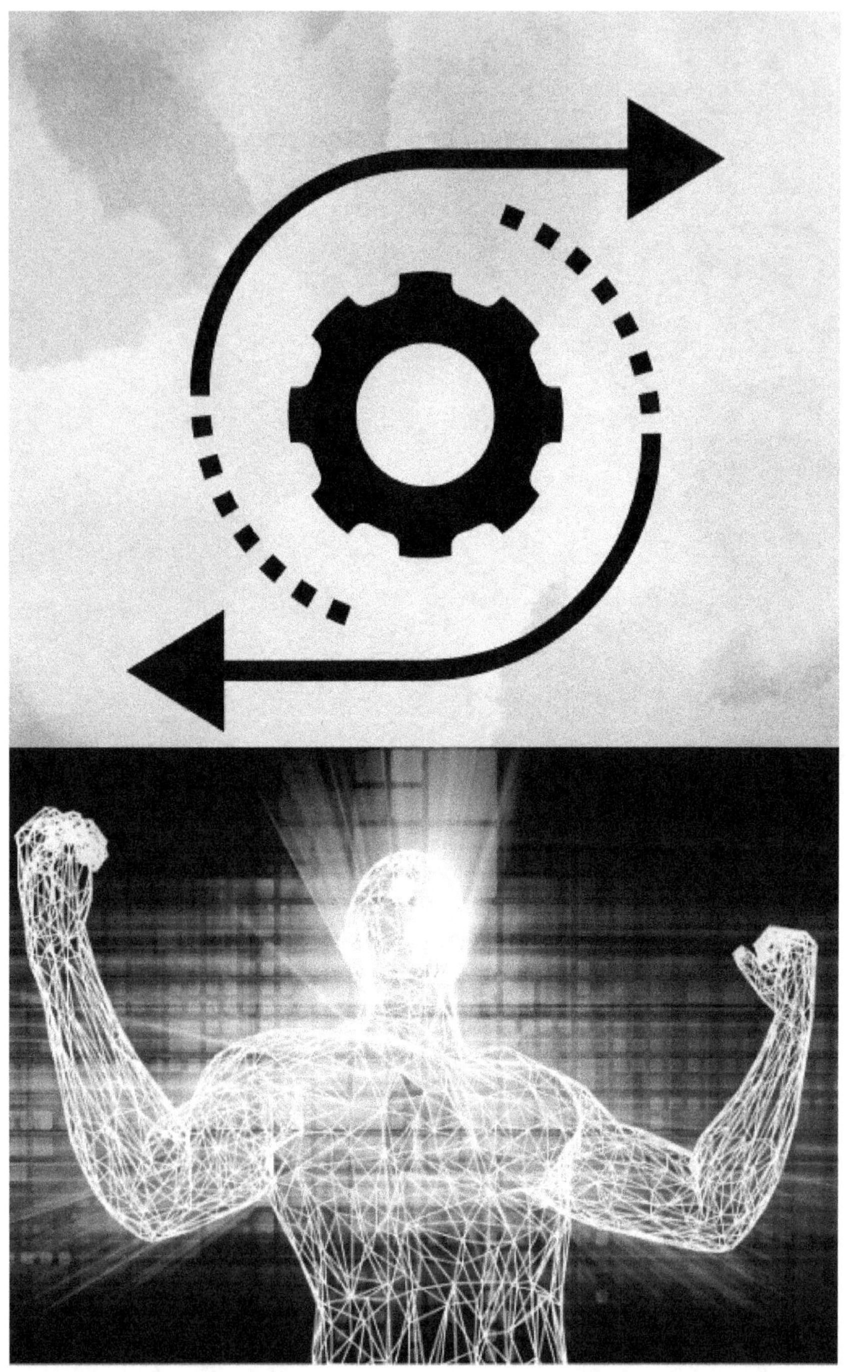

In the realm of Yoga Yin, transformation becomes an inevitable and beautiful part of the journey. This chapter explores the art of embracing change and growth through the practice of Yoga Yin. As we settle into stillness and surrender, we learn to let go of attachments and expectations, fostering a sense of openness and receptivity to the unfolding of life. By cultivating a positive outlook on life, we embrace the transformative power of Yoga Yin and discover the profound potential for inner and outer change.

Embracing Change and Growth through Yoga Yin

Change is a constant and natural aspect of life, and Yoga Yin becomes a sanctuary where we learn to flow with the currents of transformation. In the practice of stillness and surrender, we encounter the impermanence of each moment, acknowledging that life is in a constant state of flux. In Yoga Yin, we learn to embrace change and growth as an integral part of our journey. As we settle into postures, we observe how our bodies respond to the passage of time, how physical sensations come and go, and how emotions rise and fall. The practice becomes a mirror to the impermanence of life, teaching us to find comfort and ease amidst change. Through the physical practice of Yoga Yin, we also tap into the transformative power of the breath. The breath is a constant flow of inhalations and exhalations, mirroring the cycles of life and death. By breathing consciously, we connect with the ever-changing rhythm of existence, grounding us in the present moment and embracing the flow of life.

Letting Go of Attachments and Expectations

Yoga Yin becomes a practice of surrendering not only to physical sensations but also to our attachments and expectations. As we settle into postures, we may encounter mental resistance and expectations of how the practice should unfold. The practice of letting go teaches us to release these mental constructs and embrace each moment with openness and acceptance. Attachments to outcomes and expectations can hinder our ability to fully experience the present moment. By holding on to fixed ideas of how the practice should be or how life should unfold, we limit our capacity for growth and transformation. Letting go of these attachments liberates us from the constraints of the mind, allowing us to flow with the current of life with grace and ease. The practice of letting go extends beyond the mat, infusing our daily lives with a sense of freedom and lightness. By relinquishing the need for control and embracing the uncertainty of life, we open ourselves to the infinite possibilities that lie ahead.

Cultivating a Positive Outlook on Life

Yoga Yin nurtures a positive outlook on life by encouraging us to approach each moment with mindfulness and compassion. In the stillness of the practice, we learn to focus on the present moment, releasing the grip of past regrets and future anxieties. By being fully present, we cultivate a sense of gratitude for the simple joys of life. Moreover, the practice of Yoga Yin fosters self-compassion, allowing us to be kind and gentle with ourselves, even in moments of challenge. By approaching our practice with patience and acceptance, we learn to extend the same kindness to others and the world around us. A positive outlook on life does not deny the reality of difficulties and challenges. Instead, it allows us to face these obstacles with courage and resilience. In Yoga Yin, we learn that the most challenging moments are often opportunities for growth and self-discovery. Cultivating a positive outlook on life also involves nurturing an attitude of curiosity and openness. As we settle into postures with a sense of exploration, we approach life with a spirit of wonder and receptivity. This openness invites new experiences and possibilities, enriching our journey of transformation.

Embracing transformation through Yoga Yin is a profound and transformative journey of growth and self-discovery. By settling into stillness and surrender, we learn to flow with the currents of change, embracing the impermanence of each moment. The practice becomes a mirror to the cycles of life, guiding us to find comfort and ease amidst transformation. Letting go of attachments and expectations liberates us from the constraints of the mind, allowing us to embrace the uncertainty of life with openness and acceptance. By releasing the need for control, we open ourselves to the infinite possibilities that lie ahead.

Cultivating a positive outlook on life through Yoga Yin fosters mindfulness, compassion, and gratitude. By being fully present and self-compassionate, we extend kindness to ourselves and others. This positive outlook empowers us to face challenges with courage and resilience, viewing them as opportunities for growth and self-discovery.

Conclusion

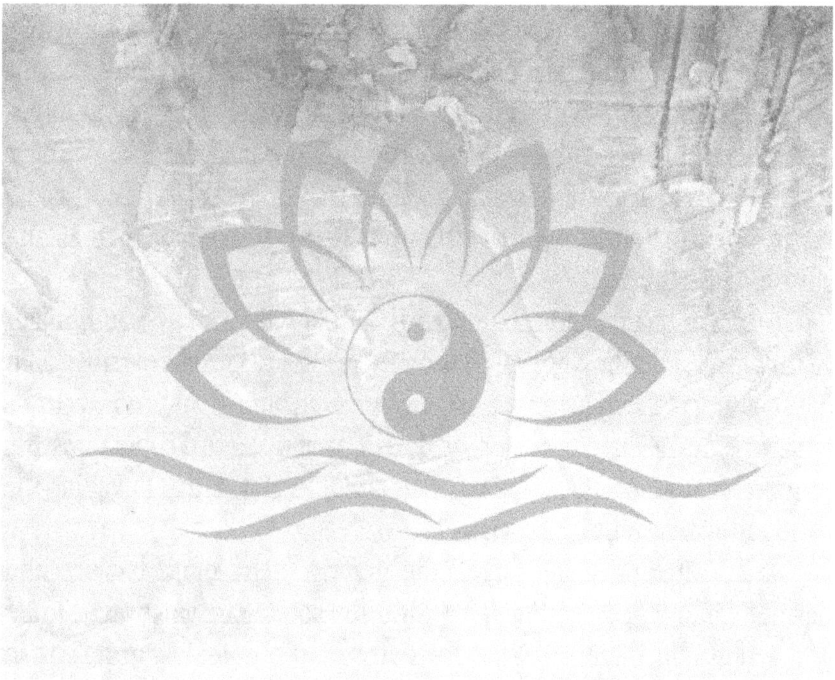

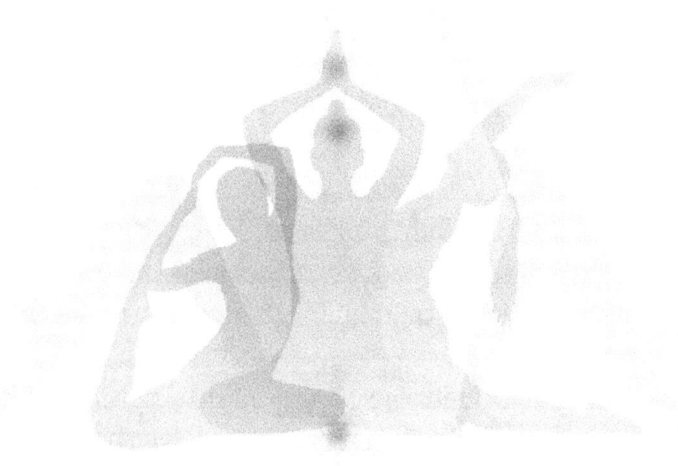

In the sanctuary of Yoga Yin, we have embarked on a transformative journey of self-discovery, inner strength, and flexibility. Throughout this book, we have explored the essence of Yoga Yin, delving into the stillness, surrender, and mindfulness that define this unique practice. We have discovered the profound interplay between the body and mind, embracing the holistic approach that nurtures our physical, mental, and emotional well-being.

Yoga Yin has gifted us with the wisdom of self-awareness, guiding us to listen to our bodies, honour our boundaries, and cultivate resilience. It has taught us to soften around discomfort, welcoming emotional release, and inviting healing into our lives. The practice of Yin postures has become a gateway to emotional balance and mental clarity, unveiling the vast landscape of our inner selves.

As we integrated Yin and Yang practices, we found balance and harmony in our lives, embracing both stillness and movement, surrender and action. The dance between the two has empowered us to flow with the rhythm of life, adapting to change with grace and ease.

In the profound journey of meditation and mindfulness, we explored the depths of our minds and hearts, uncovering the hidden treasures within. The stillness of Yoga Yin has become a fertile ground for self-discovery, healing, and personal growth, allowing us to release attachments and expectations and embrace the transformative power of the present moment.

Through the pages of this book, we have encountered the boundless potential that resides within each breath, each sensation, and each moment of surrender. The practice of Yoga Yin has become a sanctuary where we find solace and strength, guiding us toward a profound sense of self-acceptance and wholeness.

Now, I would like to invite you, dear readers, to review this book. Your feedback and insights are invaluable, and your reviews will help others discover the transformative power of Yoga Yin. If this book has touched your heart and inspired your practice, please take a moment to share your thoughts on online platforms, social media, or with friends and fellow yogis.

Your reviews will serve as a guiding light for those seeking to embark on their own journey of Yoga Yin, cultivating inner strength, flexibility, and mindfulness. Let us come together as a community, embracing the transformative potential of this practice and supporting each other on our paths of self-discovery and well-being.

In closing, I extend my deepest gratitude for joining me on this journey through the pages of Yoga Yin: Cultivating Inner Strength and Flexibility. May this practice continue to illuminate your path, guiding you toward profound self-realization, and empowering you to embrace the beauty of life's ever-unfolding dance.

With heartfelt appreciation,

Dr. Jilesh

Don't miss out!

Visit the website below and you can sign up to receive emails whenever Dr. Jilesh publishes a new book. There's no charge and no obligation.

https://books2read.com/r/B-A-BWVT-UKMMC

BOOKS2READ

Connecting independent readers to independent writers.

Also by Dr. Jilesh

Emotions

Wheel of Emotions: Balancing Emotions for Achieving Success at Work

The Art and Science of Emotions: Decoding the Secrets of the Brain

Health & Wellness

Teens Mental Health in the Social Media Era: Finding Balance in a Digital World

Mental Health Matters: A Comprehensive Guide to Mental Health Disorders

Mental Health Awareness: A Comprehensive Guide to Mental Health for Men

Mental Health Awareness: A Comprehensive Guide to Mental Health for Women

The Art of Dark Psychology: A Guide to Dark Psychology Tricks

The Mindful Child: Strategies for Nurturing Mental Growth and Child Development

Sleep Paralysis Exposed: Unmasking Its Causes and the Demonic Reality

Parenting

Boy to Man : The Mother's Guide to Raising an Extraordinary Son

Guiding Her Path: A Father's Guide to Raising a Strong Daughter

Professional Development

Gentle Leadership Unleashed: Transforming Challenges into Opportunities for Success

Emotional Intelligence Mastery: Harnessing the Power of Emotions for Personal and Professional Success

Religion and Spirituality

Journey to Infinity: The Quest for Eternal Life and the Secrets of Immortality

Spiritual Guide - Exploring Zodiac Love Compatibility For Better Relationships.

Angel Numbers: Unlocking Divine Messages

Spiritual Infusion 1111 : Exploring The Sacred Path

Twin Flame Vs Soulmate: Unveiling the Rare Twin Flame Signs and Soulmate Secrets

Gayatri Mantra: Awaken the Divine Light Within

Divine Guidance: Yes or No Tarot for Clear Direction

Maha Mrityunjaya Mantra: Awaken the Immortal Within with Sacred Vibration Frequencies

Soulful Prayers for Healing and Renewal

The Spirit Guide: Nurturing the Bond with your Spiritual Animal

A Family's Guide to Spiritual Warfare Prayers : How to protect home and family from Spiritual darkness

Spiritual Fruits - Sowing Seeds of Grace

Grace for Purpose Prayers: Empowering Your Journey
Prayers for the Guardian Angel : A Book of Prayer for Divine
Protection
Prayer for Students: A Collection of Prayers for Students Success
Prayers for Night: Seeking Guidance and Blessings in Darkness
Rays of Hope: Prayers For The Morning Grace
Divine Empowerment: Prayers for Strength and Courage

Self Help
The Subconscious Mind - Activate Your Inner MOJO
Manifesting Miracles - Daily Affirmations for Love, Happiness, and
Inner Peace
51 Little-Known Mini Meditation Techniques for Instant
Manifestation
Alchemy: A Journey of Transformation and Self-Discovery
Breaking the Darkness : A Journey of Healing and Recovery from
Depression
The Procrastination Puzzle - Breaking the Cycle and Achieving Success
The Meaning of Dreams: 7 Dreams you Should Never Ignore
Growth Mindset: A Mindset Shift Towards Limitless Possibilities
Zen in Five: Mastering the Art of 5-Minute Meditation
Chakra Healing: A Beginner's Guide to Self-Healing Techniques for
Inner Balance
Guided Meditation for Lucid Dreaming and Self-Discovery
Spiritual Psychosis: A Guide to Spiritual Psychosis for Finding Clarity
Healing Frequencies Amplified: Harnessing the Healing Power of
Vibration
Supercharge Your Life: Law of Attraction Affirmations for Wealth and
Prosperity
The Lucky Numbers Dream Guide: Discovering Your Lucky Numbers
Mindset for Success: Achieving the Sustainable Development Goals

Yoga
Brain Yoga: Yoga Practices for a Sharp Mind
Yoga Yin: Cultivating Inner Strength and Flexibility

Standalone
The Entrepreneur Mindset: Crafting a Winning and Strong Mindset

Watch for more at https://www.healingoraclewisdom.com/.